Table of Contents

Introduction
- Welcome and an overview of the eBook
- The importance of sustainable weight loss
- Setting realistic expectations

Chapter 1: Understanding Weight Loss
- The science of weight gain and loss
- Body composition and metabolism
- The role of genetics in weight management

Chapter 2: Nutrition for Sustainable Weight Loss
- The fundamentals of a balanced diet
- Macronutrients and micronutrients
- Meal planning and portion control

Chapter 3: The Power of Physical Activity
- Benefits of exercise for weight loss
- Types of physical activity
- Creating an effective workout routine

Chapter 4: Metabolism and Weight Loss
- Metabolism myths and truths
- Strategies to boost metabolism

- The impact of muscle on metabolism

Chapter 5: Behavior and Mindset
- Understanding emotional eating
- Setting SMART goals
- Mindful eating and self-control

Chapter 6: Sustainable Weight Loss Strategies
- The importance of gradual progress
- Avoiding fad diets and quick fixes
- Strategies for long-term success

Chapter 7: Meal Planning and Recipes
- Sample meal plans for different dietary preferences
- Healthy and delicious recipes for weight loss
- Portion control and mindful eating practices

Chapter 8: Monitoring and Tracking Progress
- The role of food journals
- Tracking physical activity and progress
- Adjusting strategies as needed

Chapter 9: Overcoming Plateaus and Setbacks

- Common weight loss plateaus and how to break through them
- Dealing with setbacks and staying motivated
- Seeking support and accountability

Chapter 10: Maintaining Weight Loss
- Strategies for weight maintenance
- Long-term lifestyle changes
- Celebrating successes and setting new goals

Conclusion
- Summarizing key takeaways
- Encouragement and motivation for readers
- Final thoughts and a call to action

Introduction

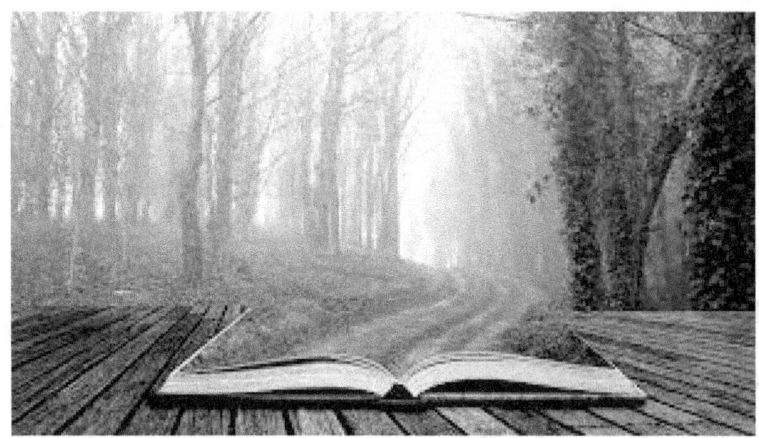

Welcome to "*The Ultimate Guide to Sustainable Weight Loss: Science-Based Strategies.*" In the pages that follow, we are about to embark on a transformative journey towards a healthier and happier you. This eBook is more than just a compilation of tips and tricks; it's your roadmap to achieving lasting weight loss success.

The Importance of Sustainable Weight Loss

Weight loss is a goal that countless individuals strive for, often in search of quick fixes and rapid results. However, the true path to improved health and well-being is not found in crash diets or extreme measures. Sustainable weight loss is the cornerstone of our journey, and it's a goal worth pursuing for numerous reasons.

Sustainable weight loss is not merely about shedding pounds but about making lasting, positive changes to your lifestyle. It's about forging a healthier relationship with food, embracing physical activity, and nurturing a mindset that supports your goals. Sustainable weight loss is the path to better overall health, increased energy, enhanced self-esteem, and a reduced risk of numerous weight-related health issues.

Setting Realistic Expectations

Before we dive into the depths of science-based weight loss strategies, it's vital to set realistic expectations. Sustainable weight loss is not a race; it's a journey. It's a process that requires time, dedication, and patience. The results you achieve should be a reflection of your individual efforts and choices, rather than conforming to unrealistic societal standards.

Throughout this eBook, we'll emphasize the importance of gradual progress, behavior change, and maintaining your achievements over time. Setting realistic expectations is about understanding that there will be both triumphs and setbacks along the way, and that's entirely normal. What's essential is your commitment to the process and your willingness to learn and adapt as you go.

So, whether you're starting your weight loss journey or seeking to revamp your existing approach, remember that this eBook is your trusted companion. We'll explore the science behind weight loss, delve into effective strategies, and equip you with the knowledge and tools you need to achieve and maintain your desired weight. Together, we'll unlock the secrets to sustainable weight loss and embark on a path towards a healthier, happier you.

Chapter 1: Understanding Weight Loss

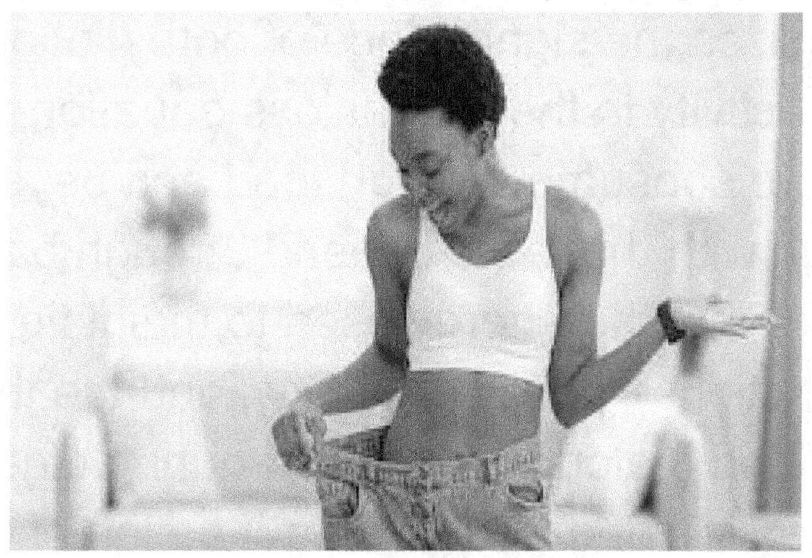

In our journey towards sustainable weight loss, it's crucial to begin with a comprehensive understanding of the science behind weight gain and loss. In this chapter, we'll delve into three fundamental aspects:

1. The Science of Weight Gain and Loss

Weight management isn't a mysterious process; it's deeply rooted in the laws of physics and biology. At its core, weight gain occurs when we consume more calories than our bodies burn, leading to an energy surplus stored as fat. Weight loss, conversely, transpires when we create an energy deficit by burning more calories than we ingest.

Understanding this calorie balance principle is vital. It emphasizes the significance of both diet and physical activity in the weight loss equation. The calories we consume through food and beverages must align with those we expend through basal metabolic rate (the energy used to maintain basic bodily functions), physical activity, and the thermic effect of food (calories expended during digestion). This understanding forms the foundation of sustainable weight loss strategies.

2. **Body Composition and Metabolism**

Body composition is the composition of the human body in terms of lean mass (muscles, bones, organs) and fat mass. A key aspect of sustainable weight loss is preserving or even increasing lean mass while reducing fat mass. Lean mass contributes significantly to a higher basal metabolic rate, which means you burn more calories at rest. This is where strength training and resistance exercises play a crucial role.

Metabolism, often a subject of fascination, is the sum of all chemical processes in the body that generate and use energy. It encompasses the basal metabolic rate and the energy expended during physical activities and digestion. While genetics influence some aspects of metabolism, lifestyle choices can also have a substantial impact. By boosting your metabolism through exercise and a well-balanced diet, you can create a more effective environment for weight loss.

3. The Role of Genetics in Weight Management

Genetics plays a role in how our bodies store and use fat, as well as our predisposition to certain weight-related conditions. Some individuals may have a genetic makeup that makes it slightly easier or harder to lose weight. However, it's essential to recognize that genetics is just one piece of the puzzle. Lifestyle factors, such as diet and physical activity, have a significant influence on weight management, and they are within our control.

Understanding your genetic predispositions can be valuable in tailoring your weight loss approach. It can help you identify potential challenges and choose strategies that are most likely to be effective for your unique genetic makeup.

In summary, this chapter has laid the groundwork for our journey towards sustainable weight loss. We've explored the fundamental principles of weight gain and loss, the significance of body composition and metabolism, and the role genetics plays in weight management. Armed with this knowledge, we are better equipped to embark on a scientifically sound weight loss adventure that will lead to lasting results.

Chapter 2: Nutrition for Sustainable Weight Loss

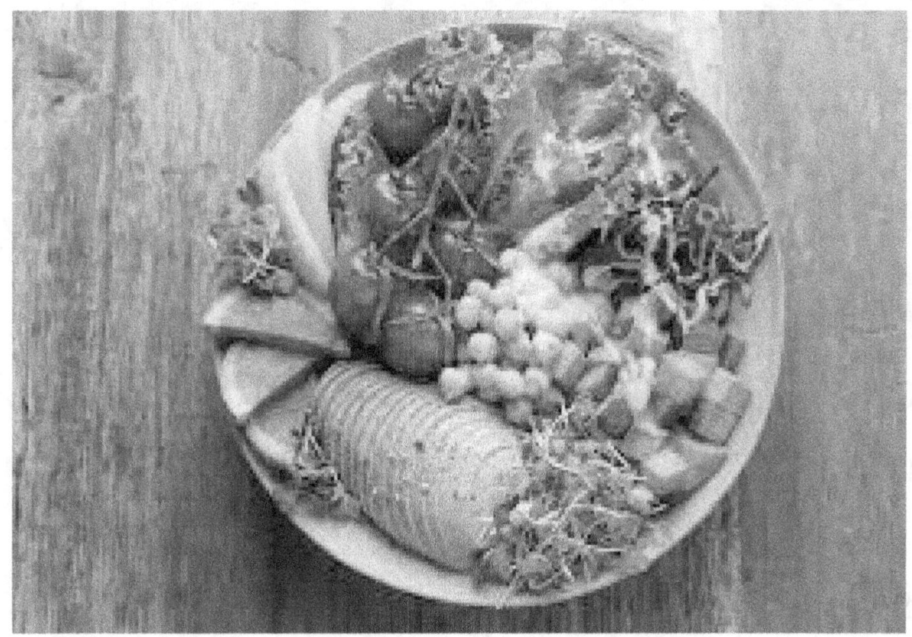

In our quest for sustainable weight loss, nutrition plays a pivotal role. This chapter explores the essential elements of a balanced diet, the significance of macronutrients and micronutrients, and strategies for effective meal planning and portion control.

The Fundamentals of a Balanced Diet

A balanced diet is the cornerstone of sustainable weight loss. It ensures that your body receives all the nutrients it needs for optimal functioning while managing your calorie intake. The key components of a balanced diet include:

- **Fruits and Vegetables**: Rich in vitamins, minerals, fiber, and antioxidants, these are essential for overall health and weight management.

- **Lean Proteins**: Lean meats, poultry, fish, tofu, and legumes are excellent sources of protein, which supports muscle growth and maintenance.

- **Whole Grains**: Incorporating whole grains like brown rice, quinoa, and whole wheat bread provides complex carbohydrates for sustained energy.

- **Healthy Fats:** Include sources of healthy fats, such as avocados, nuts, and olive oil, which are crucial for various bodily functions.

- **Dairy or Dairy Alternatives:** These provide calcium and other nutrients important for bone health.

Macronutrients and Micronutrients

Understanding the role of macronutrients (carbohydrates, proteins, and fats) and micronutrients (vitamins and minerals) is essential for effective weight management:

- **Carbohydrates**: They are the body's primary source of energy. Focus on complex carbohydrates like whole grains, fruits, and vegetables, while limiting simple sugars.

- **Proteins**: Essential for muscle growth and repair. Including lean protein sources in your diet can help you feel fuller for longer.

- **Fats**: While fats are calorie-dense, they are also important for hormone production and overall health. Choose healthy fats in moderation.

- **Vitamins and Minerals**: These micronutrients are crucial for various bodily functions. A diverse diet ensures you get the full spectrum of vitamins and minerals.

Meal Planning and Portion Control

One of the keys to sustainable weight loss is meal planning and portion control. Here are some practical tips to help you make healthier choices:

- **Portion Awareness**: Learn to recognize proper portion sizes to prevent overeating. Measuring and using smaller plates can be helpful.

- **Meal Frequency**: Focus on regular, balanced meals and snacks to maintain stable blood sugar levels and prevent excessive hunger.

- **Mindful Eating**: Pay attention to what you're eating, savor each bite, and avoid distractions like TV or your phone. This can help you eat in moderation.

- **Meal Prep**: Planning your meals in advance allows you to make healthier choices and avoid impulsive, less nutritious options.

- **Hydration**: Drinking enough water is essential for overall health and can help control appetite. Sometimes thirst is mistaken for hunger.

By mastering the fundamentals of a balanced diet, understanding macronutrients and micronutrients, and practicing meal planning and portion control, you'll be better equipped to make informed dietary choices that support your weight loss journey. The knowledge and strategies presented in this chapter lay a solid foundation for your path to sustainable weight loss.

Chapter 3: The Power of Physical Activity

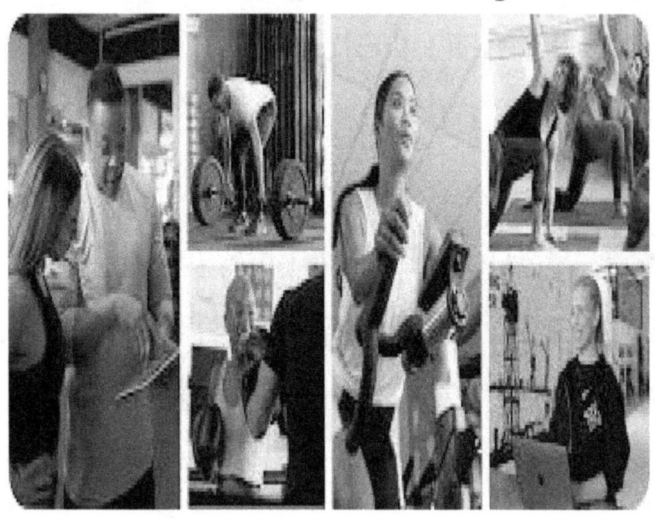

In our pursuit of sustainable weight loss, physical activity stands as a formidable ally. This chapter explores the manifold benefits of exercise for weight loss, introduces various types of physical activity, and guides you in creating an effective workout routine.

Benefits of Exercise for Weight Loss

Exercise isn't just about burning calories; it offers a plethora of advantages for those seeking to shed excess weight:

- **Calorie Expenditure**: Physical activity increases your energy expenditure, creating a calorie deficit essential for weight loss.

- **Metabolism Boost**: Regular exercise elevates your resting metabolic rate, helping you burn more calories even when at rest.

- **Muscle Preservation**: Exercise, particularly resistance training, helps preserve lean muscle mass during weight loss, which is vital for a higher metabolism.

- **Appetite Regulation**: Physical activity can assist in controlling appetite and reducing cravings.

- **Mood and Motivation**: Exercise releases endorphins, improving mood and motivation, which can be instrumental in adhering to a weight loss plan.

Types of Physical Activity

Exercise doesn't come in a one-size-fits-all package. There are various forms of physical activity, allowing you to choose what aligns with your preferences and lifestyle:

- **Aerobic Exercises**: Activities like running, swimming, and cycling boost cardiovascular fitness and contribute to calorie burning.

- **Strength Training**: Resistance exercises with weights or bodyweight (e.g., push-ups) help build and maintain muscle mass.

- **Flexibility and Mobility Work**: Yoga and stretching exercises enhance flexibility, aiding overall body function.

- **High-Intensity Interval Training (HIIT):** HIIT workouts involve short, intense bursts of exercise followed by brief rest periods, resulting in efficient calorie burning.

- **Sport and Recreation**: Engaging in sports and recreational activities can make exercise enjoyable and less like a chore.

Creating an Effective Workout Routine

Building an effective workout routine requires careful planning and consideration of your goals and preferences:

- **Goal Setting**: Define your fitness and weight loss objectives. Do you aim to lose a specific amount of weight, build muscle, or enhance overall fitness?

- **Frequency**: Determine how many days per week you can commit to exercise. Aim for a balance of cardiovascular, strength, and flexibility training.

- **Duration and Intensity**: Decide how long each session will be and at what intensity level. Gradually increase the intensity as you progress.

- **Variety**: Incorporate a mix of activities to prevent boredom and work different muscle groups.

- **Rest and Recovery**: Allow your body adequate time to recover between workouts to prevent overuse injuries.

- **Professional Guidance**: If you're new to exercise or have specific goals, consider consulting a fitness professional for guidance.

By harnessing the benefits of exercise, exploring diverse types of physical activity, and crafting an effective workout routine, you'll be on the path to sustainable weight loss. Remember, the journey is unique to you, and consistency and enjoyment are key factors in your long-term success.

Chapter 4: Metabolism and Weight Loss

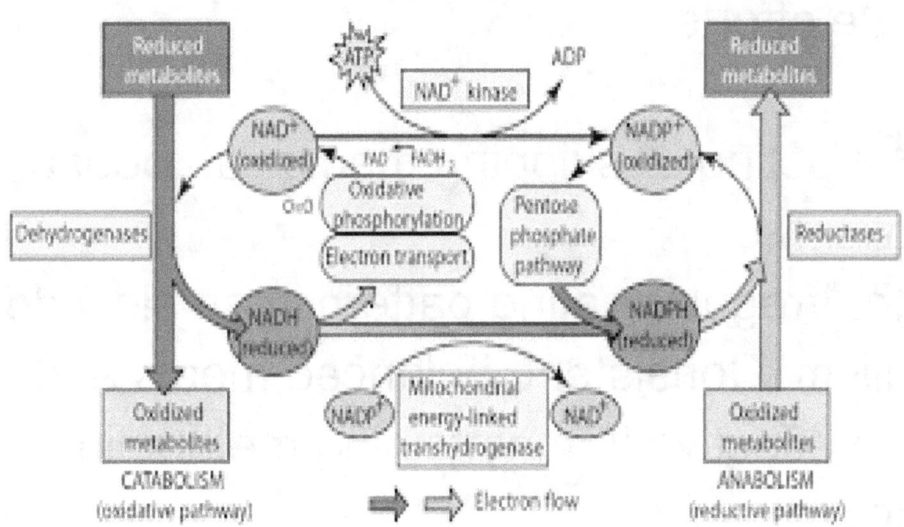

In our journey towards sustainable weight loss, understanding metabolism is pivotal. This chapter delves into the common myths and truths surrounding metabolism, strategies to boost your metabolic rate, and the profound impact of muscle on metabolism.

Metabolism Myths and Truths

Metabolism is a topic that's often shrouded in myths. Let's dispel some of the common misconceptions:

Myth 1: Metabolism is fixed and unchangeable.
   - Truth: Metabolism can be influenced by various factors, including age, genetics, and lifestyle

choices. It's not static and can be modified through deliberate efforts.

Myth 2: Fasting or skipping meals can boost metabolism.
   - Truth: Irregular eating patterns can slow down metabolism. Consistent, balanced meals and snacks are more effective in maintaining metabolic efficiency.

Myth 3: Certain foods have "negative" calories.
   - Truth: While some foods have low calorie density, the concept of negative calories is an oversimplification. All foods have calories, and the focus should be on the overall quality of your diet.

Strategies to Boost Metabolism

Elevating your metabolism can enhance your body's ability to burn calories efficiently. Consider these strategies:

- **Strength Training**: Engage in resistance exercises to build and maintain muscle. Muscle tissue requires more energy at rest than fat, increasing your resting metabolic rate.

- **High-Intensity Interval Training (HIIT)**: HIIT workouts can significantly increase calorie burning and stimulate metabolism for hours post-exercise.

- **Adequate Protein Intake**: Include sufficient protein in your diet to support muscle preservation and a higher thermic effect of food.

- **Balanced Nutrition**: Consume a well-balanced diet to ensure your body has the nutrients it needs for optimal metabolic function.

- **Hydration**: Staying well-hydrated is essential for efficient metabolic processes.

- **Adequate Sleep**: Quality sleep is crucial for metabolic health. Poor sleep can disrupt hormones that regulate appetite and energy expenditure.

The Impact of Muscle on Metabolism

Muscle plays a pivotal role in the metabolic rate of the body. Here's why:

- **Resting Metabolic Rate (RMR):** Muscle tissue is more metabolically active than fat tissue. Therefore, individuals with a higher proportion of muscle have a higher RMR, meaning they burn more calories at rest.

- **Thermic Effect of Food (TEF):** The process of digesting and absorbing nutrients burns calories. Protein has the highest thermic effect, and consuming it can slightly boost metabolism.

- **Physical Activity**: Muscle is crucial for various physical activities. The more muscle you have, the more efficiently you can engage in exercise and burn calories.

By understanding metabolism myths and truths, employing strategies to boost metabolism, and recognizing the substantial impact of muscle on metabolism, you gain insights into how to harness your body's natural mechanisms to support sustainable weight loss. Embracing these principles empowers you to make informed choices that contribute to your long-term success.

Chapter 5: Behavior and Mindset

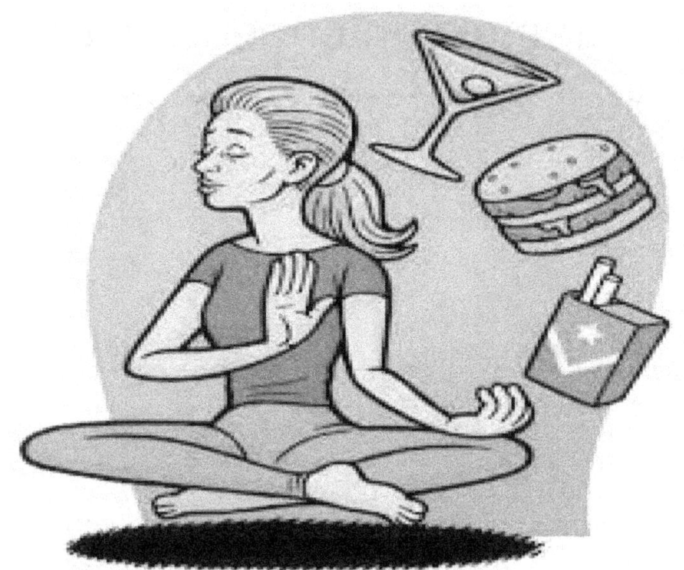

The journey to sustainable weight loss is not solely about what you eat and how much you exercise; it's also about understanding your behaviors and cultivating a positive mindset. In this chapter, we explore the critical aspects of understanding emotional eating, setting SMART goals, and practicing mindful eating and self-control.

Understanding Emotional Eating

Emotional eating is a significant challenge for many individuals on a weight loss journey. It involves using food as a way to cope with or alleviate emotions, such as stress, sadness, or boredom. Recognizing and addressing emotional eating is crucial for lasting success:

- **Identification**: Learn to recognize when you're eating in response to emotions rather than physical hunger. Keep a food journal to track your eating patterns.

- **Alternative Coping Strategies**: Instead of turning to food, explore other coping mechanisms like exercise, meditation, or engaging in hobbies.

- **Mindfulness**: Practice being present in the moment, acknowledging your emotions without judgment, and choosing how to respond rather than react.

Setting SMART Goals

Effective goal-setting is a cornerstone of sustainable weight loss. **SMART** goals are *Specific*, *Measurable*, *Achievable*, *Relevant*, and *Time-bound*. Here's how to apply this framework to your weight loss goals:

- **Specific**: Define clear, precise objectives. Instead of saying, "I want to lose weight," specify how much weight you want to lose and in what time frame.

- **Measurable**: Goals should be quantifiable. Use numbers and metrics to track your progress.

- **Achievable**: Ensure your goals are realistic and attainable. Unrealistic goals can lead to frustration and disappointment.

- **Relevant**: Your goals should align with your values and your overarching desire for a healthier lifestyle.

- **Time-bound**: Set deadlines for your goals. This creates a sense of urgency and commitment.

Mindful Eating and Self-Control

Mindful eating involves being fully present while you eat, paying attention to your body's hunger and fullness cues, and savoring each bite. It helps foster a healthy relationship with food and enhances self-control:

- **Portion Awareness**: Serve smaller portions and savor each bite, allowing your body to recognize fullness.

- **Slow Down**: Eating slowly gives your brain time to process signals of fullness, reducing the risk of overeating.

- **Remove Distractions**: Avoid eating in front of the TV or computer. Focus on your meal and enjoy it without distractions.

- **Emotional Awareness**: Be attuned to emotional triggers for overeating. When emotions arise, practice self-awareness and consider alternative ways to address them.

Cultivating a positive mindset, recognizing and managing emotional eating, setting SMART goals, and practicing mindful eating are key components of the behavioral and psychological aspects of sustainable weight loss. By incorporating these principles into your journey, you'll gain greater control over your habits and mindset, ultimately contributing to long-term success.

Chapter 6: Sustainable Weight Loss Strategies

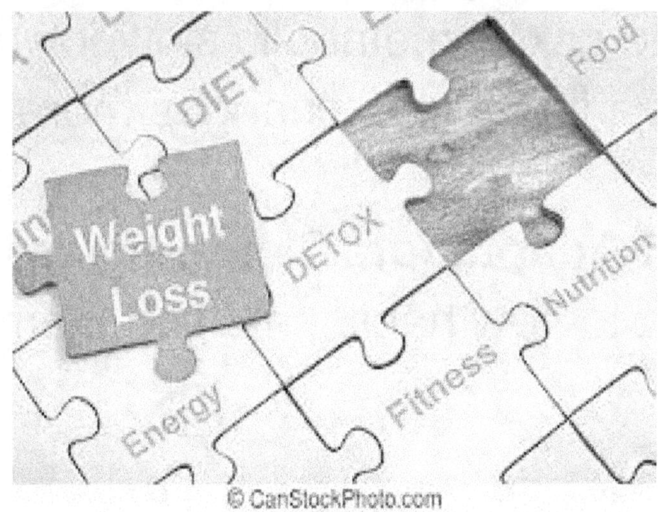

© CanStockPhoto.com

Sustainable weight loss is not about quick fixes or temporary solutions; it's about adopting a lifestyle that promotes lasting well-being. In this chapter, we explore the significance of gradual progress, the pitfalls of fad diets and quick fixes, and strategies for long-term success.

The Importance of Gradual Progress

One of the key principles of sustainable weight loss is gradual progress. Rather than striving for dramatic, short-term changes, a slow and steady approach offers several advantages:

- **Maintaining Metabolism**: Gradual weight loss minimizes the risk of metabolic slowdown, allowing your body to adjust to the changes more effectively.

- **Behavioral Adaptation**: Slow progress gives you time to adapt to new habits, making them more likely to stick.

- **Sustainability**: Gradual changes are easier to incorporate into your daily life, promoting long-term adherence.

- **Healthier Mindset**: Focusing on small, achievable goals fosters a positive mindset and reduces the likelihood of discouragement.

Avoiding Fad Diets and Quick Fixes

Fad diets and quick fixes may promise rapid results, but they often come with detrimental consequences for your long-term well-being. Here's why it's essential to steer clear of them:

- **Nutritional Deficiencies**: Fad diets can lack essential nutrients, potentially leading to health issues.

- **Unrealistic Expectations**: They often create unsustainable expectations, setting you up for disappointment and yo-yo dieting.

- **Loss of Lean Mass**: Quick fixes often result in muscle loss, which can harm your metabolism and overall health.

- **Short-Lived Results**: Rapid weight loss is frequently short-lived, with weight regain being common.

Strategies for Long-Term Success

Sustainable weight loss is a marathon, not a sprint. To achieve and maintain your desired weight, consider these strategies:

- **Lifestyle Changes**: Focus on lasting lifestyle changes rather than short-term fixes. Gradually integrate healthier habits into your daily routine.

- **Behavior Modification**: Work on understanding and altering your eating and exercise behaviors. Seek support from professionals if needed.

- **Accountability**: Consider enlisting a support system, such as a registered dietitian, personal trainer, or a weight loss group, to hold you accountable.

- **Regular Monitoring**: Keep track of your progress, whether it's through regular weigh-ins, food journals, or fitness logs.

- **Self-Compassion**: Be kind to yourself throughout your journey. Understand that setbacks are normal, and they don't define your ultimate success.

- **Goal Revision**: As you make progress, periodically review and adjust your goals to ensure they remain relevant and motivating.

Sustainable weight loss is an ongoing commitment to your health and well-being. By embracing gradual progress, steering clear of fad diets and quick fixes, and applying these strategies for long-term success, you'll be well-prepared to achieve your weight loss goals and maintain them over time. Remember, it's not just about losing weight; it's about embracing a healthier way of life.

Chapter 7: Meal Planning and Recipes

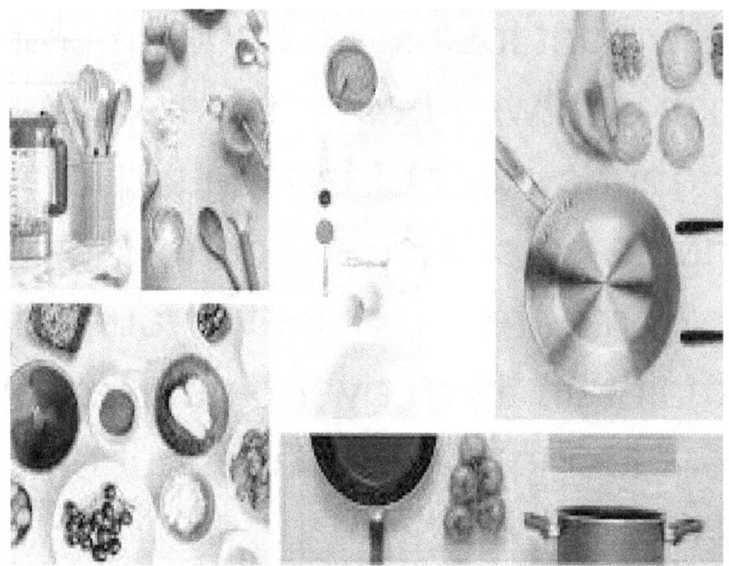

In the pursuit of sustainable weight loss, meal planning and recipes take center stage. This chapter provides sample meal plans catering to different dietary preferences, offers a selection of healthy and delicious recipes designed for weight loss, and emphasizes the importance of portion control and mindful eating practices.

Sample Meal Plans for Different Dietary Preferences

Meal planning is a key component of sustainable weight loss. Here are sample meal plans to accommodate various dietary preferences:

- **Balanced Diet Plan**: A typical day could include a breakfast of whole-grain oatmeal with berries and nuts, a lunch of mixed greens with grilled chicken, and a dinner of baked salmon with quinoa and steamed vegetables.

- **Low-Carb Diet Plan**: A low-carb day might involve scrambled eggs with spinach for breakfast, a salad with grilled shrimp for lunch, and a dinner of roasted cauliflower and broiled fish.

- **Vegetarian or Vegan Diet Plan**: Consider a day with a breakfast smoothie with almond milk, a lunch of chickpea and vegetable stir-fry, and a dinner featuring a quinoa and black bean salad.

- **Mediterranean Diet Plan:** Embrace the Mediterranean approach with a breakfast of Greek yogurt and honey, a lunch of a hummus and vegetable wrap, and a dinner featuring grilled chicken with a side of tabbouleh.

Healthy and Delicious Recipes for Weight Loss

These recipes combine flavor and nutrition, making your weight loss journey enjoyable:

- **Zucchini Noodles with Pesto**: Replace pasta with spiralized zucchini and top it with a homemade basil pesto for a low-calorie, flavorful meal.

- **Spicy Chickpea and Quinoa Bowl:** A savory blend of chickpeas, quinoa, roasted vegetables, and a spicy tahini sauce.

- **Baked Salmon with Dill Sauce**: A protein-packed dish rich in omega-3 fatty acids, served with a refreshing dill sauce.

- **Stuffed Bell Peppers**: Bell peppers filled with lean ground turkey, brown rice, and a tomato-based sauce, then baked to perfection.

- **Berry and Spinach Smoothie**: A nutrient-rich breakfast option combining spinach, berries, Greek yogurt, and a touch of honey for sweetness.

Portion Control and Mindful Eating Practices

Successful weight loss isn't just about what you eat; it's also about how you eat. Incorporating portion control and mindful eating practices can make a significant difference:

- **Use Smaller Plates**: Smaller plates can visually trick your brain into thinking you've had a larger portion.

- **Chew Slowly**: Take your time to savor each bite, and put your fork down between bites to avoid rushing through meals.

- **Pay Attention to Hunger and Fullness**: Eat when you're hungry, and stop when you're satisfied. Recognizing your body's cues is integral to mindful eating.

- **Avoid Distractions**: Turn off the TV and put away electronic devices while eating. Focus on the flavors and textures of your food.

- **Mindful Meal Prep**: Prepare meals in a mindful, deliberate manner. Consider the colors, textures, and aromas of the ingredients.

By incorporating these meal plans and recipes tailored to various dietary preferences, and by practicing portion control and mindful eating, you'll not only nourish your body but also make the weight loss journey a pleasurable and sustainable one. Meal planning, coupled with mindfulness, can be a powerful tool in achieving your weight loss goals.

Chapter 8: Monitoring and Tracking Progress

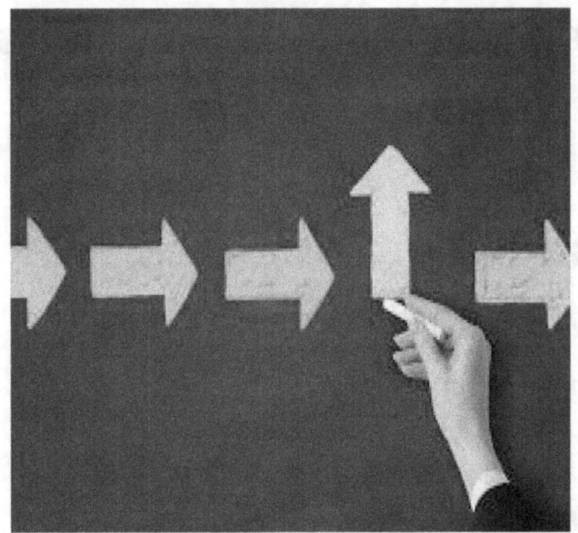

In the pursuit of sustainable weight loss, monitoring and tracking your progress are vital aspects of achieving long-term success. This chapter delves into the role of food journals, the importance of tracking physical activity and progress, and how to make necessary adjustments to your strategies as you journey towards your goals.

The Role of Food Journals

Food journals are invaluable tools for maintaining awareness of your dietary habits. Here's how they can aid in your weight loss journey:

- **Self-Reflection**: Recording what you eat encourages self-awareness and can help you identify patterns and triggers related to eating.

- **Calorie Management**: A food journal allows you to tally your daily calorie intake, ensuring you stay within your target range.

- **Accountability**: Knowing that you must document your choices can motivate you to make healthier decisions.

- **Feedback and Adjustments**: By reviewing your journal, you can pinpoint areas for improvement and adjust your meal plans accordingly.

Tracking Physical Activity and Progress

Just as monitoring food intake is crucial, keeping tabs on physical activity and progress is equally important:

- **Exercise Logs**: Document your workouts, noting the type, duration, and intensity. This information helps you track your fitness improvements.

- **Progress Photos**: Regularly take photos to visually document your journey. These photos can serve as powerful motivators.

- **Body Measurements**: In addition to the scale, measure your waist, hips, and other key areas to track physical changes more accurately.

- **Fitness Assessments**: Periodically assess your strength, flexibility, and endurance to gauge improvements.

- **Goal Progress**: Continuously assess your advancement toward your weight loss goals. Celebrate small achievements along the way.

Adjusting Strategies as Needed

No weight loss plan is static, and adjustments are often necessary for success:

- **Review and Reflect**: Periodically evaluate your food journal, exercise logs, and progress photos to identify trends and areas that require change.

- **Plateaus**: If you hit a weight loss plateau, consider adjusting your calorie intake, exercise routine, or meal composition to kickstart progress.

- **Set New Goals**: As you achieve your initial goals, set new, challenging objectives to keep your motivation high.

- **Seek Professional Guidance**: Consult a registered dietitian or fitness expert for personalized advice and strategies.

- **Stay Adaptable**: Understand that your journey may encounter setbacks or detours, and adaptability is key. Maintain your determination and flexibility in the face of challenges.

By using food journals to enhance self-awareness, tracking physical activity and progress for motivation and accountability, and making necessary adjustments to your strategies, you'll be well-equipped to overcome hurdles and stay on the path to sustainable weight loss. Remember that your journey is unique, and the ability to adapt and persevere is fundamental to achieving and maintaining your desired weight.

Chapter 9: Overcoming Plateaus and Setbacks

In the journey toward sustainable weight loss, it's common to encounter plateaus and setbacks. This chapter addresses the challenges associated with weight loss plateaus and setbacks and provides strategies for breaking through them, staying motivated, and seeking the support and accountability needed to continue your progress.

Common Weight Loss Plateaus and How to Break Through Them

Weight loss plateaus are periods when your progress stalls, and the scale seems unyielding. Understanding and addressing these plateaus are essential for your long-term success. Common strategies to overcome plateaus include:

- **Change Up Your Routine:** Alter your exercise regimen or adjust your diet by varying your food choices and meal timings.

- **Increase Physical Activity**: Add extra workout sessions or boost the intensity to increase calorie burn.

- **Review Your Eating Habits**: Reevaluate your portion sizes and the quality of the foods you consume.

- **Monitor Your Progress**: Tracking changes in body measurements, such as waist circumference or body fat percentage, can provide a more comprehensive view of your progress beyond the scale.

- **Stay Patient and Persistent**: Plateaus are a natural part of the weight loss process. Maintain your commitment and realize that progress might not always be linear.

Dealing with Setbacks and Staying Motivated

Setbacks are common and can include overeating, missed workouts, or moments of low motivation. How you deal with these setbacks can impact your journey:

- **Practice Self-Compassion**: Understand that everyone has setbacks. Instead of self-criticism, focus on self-compassion and learn from the experience.

- **Reset and Refocus**: When a setback occurs, take a moment to reset your mindset and refocus on your goals. Don't dwell on past mistakes.

- **Motivation Boosters**: Rediscover your motivation by revisiting your reasons for wanting to lose weight. Set new goals and remind yourself of the positive changes you've experienced.

- **Celebrate Small Wins**: Recognize and celebrate your achievements, even if they are not related to the number on the scale. Every small step counts.

- **Seek Inspiration**: Find inspiration from others who have overcome setbacks and achieved their goals. Success stories can provide motivation during challenging times.

Seeking Support and Accountability

Having a support system and accountability mechanisms in place can make a substantial difference in your weight loss journey:

- **Accountability Partner:** Partnering with a friend or family member who shares your goals can provide mutual support and encouragement.

- **Professional Guidance**: Consider consulting a registered dietitian, personal trainer, or therapist to guide you through challenging periods.

- **Support Groups**: Joining a weight loss or fitness group can provide a sense of community, shared experiences, and additional motivation.

- **Online Communities**: Engage with online forums or social media groups focused on weight loss and fitness. These communities offer a virtual support network.

- **Regular Check-Ins:** Establish regular check-in points with your support system to discuss your progress, setbacks, and adjustments to your plan.

Overcoming plateaus and setbacks is an integral part of your weight loss journey. By understanding and applying strategies to break through plateaus, managing setbacks, staying motivated, and seeking support and accountability, you'll be better prepared to persevere through the challenging moments and continue your path to sustainable weight loss. Remember, setbacks do not define your journey, but your commitment to overcoming them shapes your success.

Chapter 10: Maintaining Weight Loss

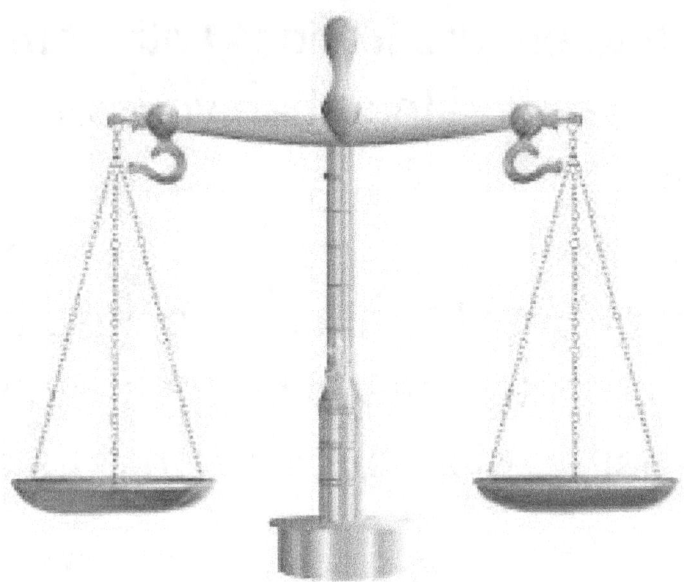

Achieving weight loss is an admirable accomplishment, but maintaining it over the long term is equally important. This final chapter discusses strategies for weight maintenance, the necessity of long-term lifestyle changes, and the importance of celebrating successes while setting new goals to continue your journey towards lasting well-being.

Strategies for Weight Maintenance

Maintaining your weight loss is a distinct phase of your journey. It requires ongoing commitment and attention to key strategies, including:

- **Calorie Management**: Continue monitoring your calorie intake to ensure it aligns with your maintenance needs rather than your weight loss requirements.

- **Regular Exercise**: Maintain a consistent exercise routine, which contributes to both physical and mental well-being. Mix up your workouts to prevent boredom.

- **Mindful Eating**: Keep practicing mindful eating to ensure you remain attuned to your body's hunger and fullness cues.

- **Occasional Checks**: Periodically monitor your weight, body measurements, and overall health to catch and address any changes early.

- **Healthy Support System**: Maintain your support network and continue seeking professional advice when needed.

Long-Term Lifestyle Changes

The transition from weight loss to maintenance necessitates the solidification of the healthy lifestyle changes you've adopted. Make these changes a permanent part of your life:

- **Balanced Diet**: Continue to enjoy a diverse, balanced diet. Remember that it's not a temporary phase but an enduring way of eating.

- **Regular Physical Activity**: Exercise should be a consistent aspect of your daily life. Find activities you genuinely enjoy and look forward to.

- **Stress Management**: Stress can impact your weight. Engage in stress-reduction practices like meditation, mindfulness, or yoga.

- **Quality Sleep**: Prioritize good sleep patterns to support your overall health and maintain optimal hormonal balance.

- **Mindset and Resilience**: Strengthen your mental resilience to face challenges and setbacks with a positive attitude.

Celebrating Successes and Setting New Goals

Recognize and celebrate your achievements on your weight loss journey. Whether you've reached your initial goal or maintained your weight loss for a significant period, it's vital to acknowledge your success:

- **Reflect on Progress**: Take time to reflect on how far you've come, what you've learned, and how your health and well-being have improved.

- **Set New Goals**: Weight maintenance is not the end of your journey. Consider setting new goals related to fitness, wellness, or other personal aspirations.

- **Celebrate Achievements**: Celebrate your successes and treat yourself to something that aligns with your new healthy lifestyle, such as a fitness-related reward.

- **Share Your Success**: Sharing your success with friends and family can be motivating, and it may inspire others to embark on their own journeys.

- **Stay Accountable**: Keep yourself accountable for maintaining your achievements, and regularly revisit and revise your goals.

Remember, maintaining weight loss is a lifelong endeavor. By implementing strategies for weight maintenance, embedding long-term lifestyle changes, celebrating your successes, and setting new goals, you'll continue your journey towards a healthier, happier, and more sustainable you. Embrace the knowledge and practices you've gained on this journey to make lasting well-being a permanent part of your life.

Conclusion

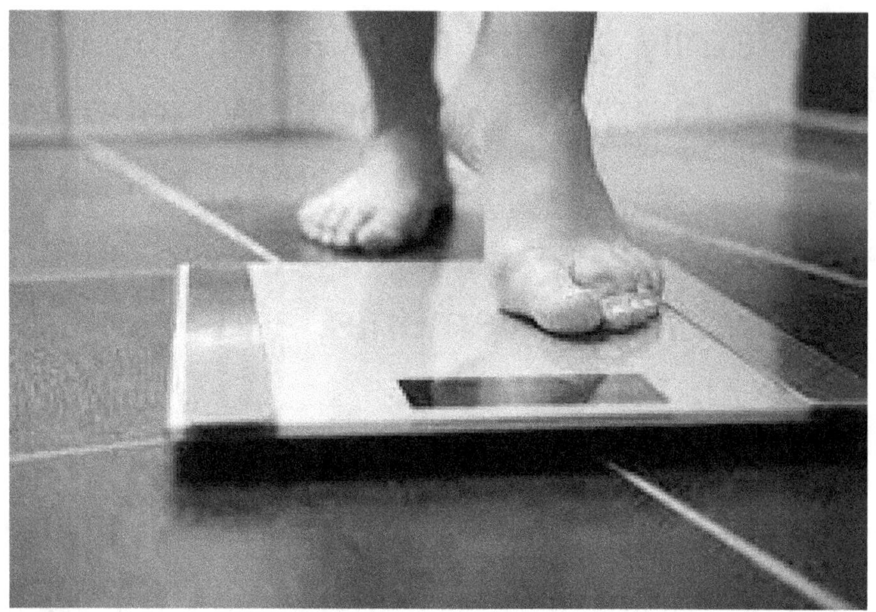

Congratulations on reaching the end of "*The Ultimate Guide to Sustainable Weight Loss*: Science-Based Strategies." Your commitment to improving your health and well-being is commendable. In this concluding chapter, we will recap key takeaways, provide encouragement and motivation, and offer some final thoughts to empower you on your weight loss journey.

Key Takeaways

Throughout this ebook, we've explored an array of science-based strategies for sustainable weight loss. Here are some of the key takeaways:

- Sustainable weight loss is about adopting a lifestyle that supports your long-term well-being.

- Understanding the science of weight gain and loss, the role of genetics, and body composition is essential for informed decision-making.

- Nutrition is a cornerstone of your journey, focusing on balanced meals, macronutrients, micronutrients, portion control, and mindful eating.

- Physical activity is a powerful ally in weight loss, with a variety of exercise types and effective workout routines at your disposal.

- Metabolism plays a crucial role in weight management, and muscle mass significantly impacts metabolic rate.

- Your behaviors, mindset, and emotional relationship with food are equally crucial for success.

- Meal planning, recipes, portion control, and mindful eating practices all contribute to a balanced and enjoyable approach to eating.

- Monitoring and tracking your progress are fundamental for ongoing success, along with strategies for overcoming plateaus and setbacks.

- Weight maintenance requires ongoing commitment to healthy lifestyle changes.

Encouragement and Motivation

Remember, the journey to sustainable weight loss is not always straightforward. It's filled with ups and downs, challenges, and victories. But every step you take, no matter how small, brings you closer to your goals. Stay motivated by:

- Celebrating your successes, no matter how modest, as they are all milestones on your path to well-being.

- Embracing the support of friends, family, and professionals who are there to guide and encourage you.

- Recognizing that setbacks are natural and should not deter you. They are opportunities for growth.

- Maintaining a positive mindset, practicing self-compassion, and believing in your ability to achieve your goals.

- Setting new goals and aspirations to continue evolving on your health and wellness journey.

Final Thoughts and a Call to Action

Your journey to sustainable weight loss is a lifelong commitment to your health and well-being. Embrace it with the knowledge that small, consistent changes can lead to significant transformations. Remember that your path is unique, and there is no one-size-fits-all approach. Make choices that align with your values and preferences, and don't be afraid to seek professional guidance when needed.

Now, it's time for your call to action. As you close this book, consider what your next steps will be. Set new goals, revisit your motivation, and take the first step towards a healthier, happier, and more sustainable you. You have all the tools and knowledge to make this journey a successful one. The road ahead may have challenges, but with determination, support, and the strategies you've learned, you're well on your way to achieving your goals and maintaining them for life. Here's to your vibrant future, filled with well-being, health, and happiness.